Breakfast for Families

Best Breakfast Recipes Made Simple

Kim C. Starling

Sommario

Introduction

The Ninja Foodi multi-cooker is just one of the devices that every person need to have in their kitchen area. The device can change four tiny tools: slow-moving cooker, air fryer, pressure cooker and also dehydrator.

This cookbook includes several of the recipes we have attempted with the multi-cooker. The dishes range from breakfast, side meals, chicken, pork, soups, fish and shellfish, treats, as well as pasta. On top of that, we have actually assembled lots of vegetarian recipes you ought to attempt. We produced these recipes considering beginners which's why the cooking procedure is methodical. Besides, the dishes are scrumptious, take pleasure in reading.

Introduction

BREAKFAST and BRUNCH

Scrambled Eggs

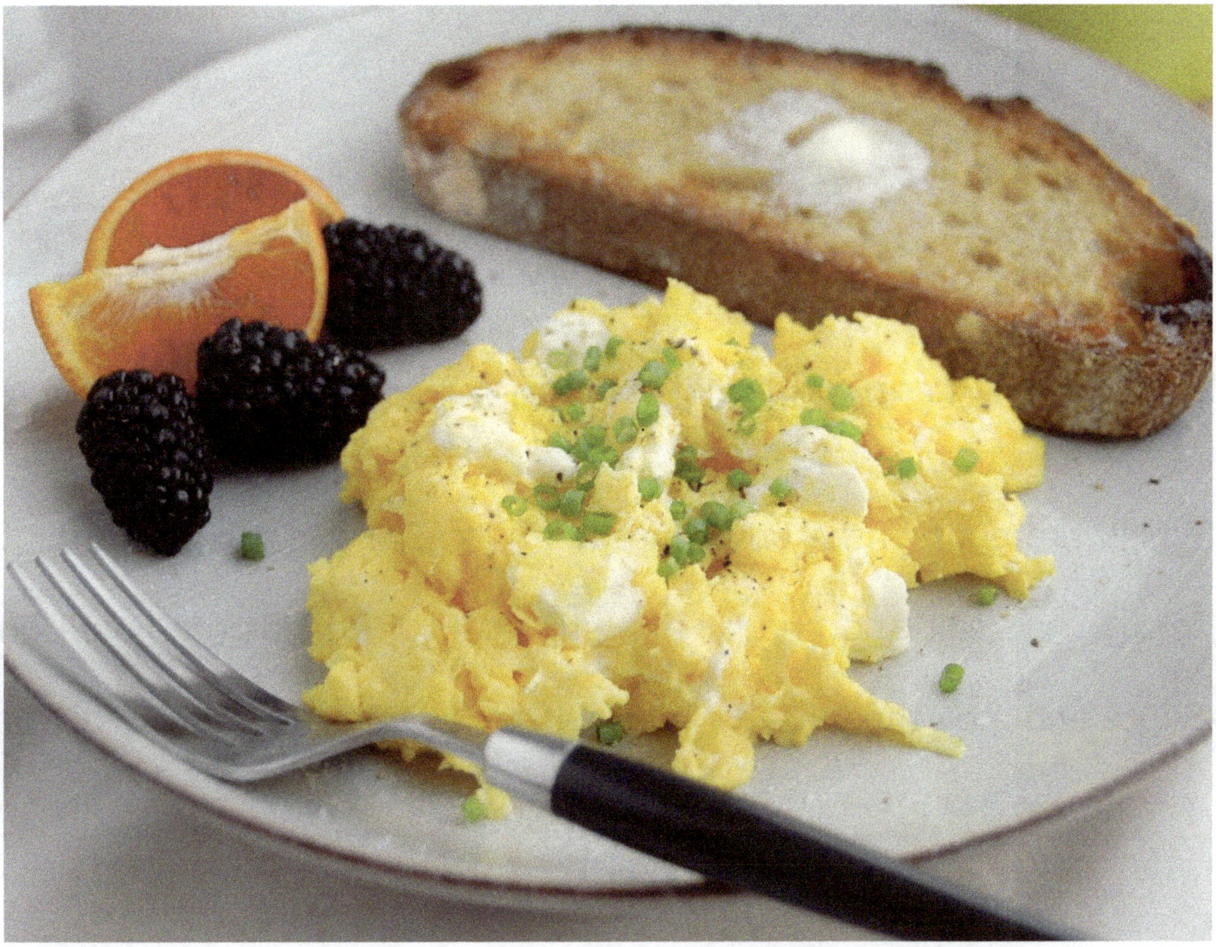

INGREDIENTS (2 Servings)

¼ cup of milk

4 whole eggs, beaten

1 tablespoon of butter

Pepper and salt

DIRECTIONS (PREP + COOK TIME: 8 MINUTES)

Whisk the eggs in the bowl and add milk. Stir the mixture until it froths. Add salt and pepper and stir again. Preheat the Foodi on Sauté and melt the butter. Add the frothed eggs and stir. Cook for 3 minutes.

Breakfast Casserole

INGREDIENTS (6 Servings)

3 cups of hash browns

1/2 lb of ground turkey-breakfast sausage

6 eggs 1/2 cup of milk

1/4 teaspoon of black pepper

1/2 teaspoon of kosher salt

1 cup of shredded Colby cheese

DIRECTIONS (PREP + COOK TIME: 30 MINUTES)

Brown the sausages on sauté mode and transfer them to a bowl. Add a cup of water to the Ninja pot and insert the reversible rack. Combine the eggs with milk, salt and pepper in the bowl. Grease the baking dish lightly and add the hash browns. Put the browned sausages into the dish and pour the egg mix over it. Sprinkle the shredded cheese over the mixture and cover it with the aluminum foil. Place the baking dish on the rack and close the crisping lid. Choose the bake/roast function and set the temperature to 375°F. Set the cooking time to 15 minutes and remember to check its progress frequently.

Bacon Veggies Combo

INGREDIENTS (4 Servings)

4 bacon slices

1 green bell pepper, seeded and chopped

1/2 cup of Monterey jack cheese

1 tablespoon of mayonnaise, preferably avocado Sautéed corn

2 scallions, chopped

DIRECTIONS (PREP + COOK TIME: 35 MINUTES)

Place the bacon slices into the basket and put it in the pot. Add the mayonnaise on top and add corn, sweet peppers, scallions, and cheese. Close the crisping lid and select the bake/roast function. Cook with a temperature of 365F for 25 minutes. Serve your combo hot.

Polenta Breakfast

INGREDIENTS (6 Servings)

1 1/2 glasses of polenta flour

1 teaspoon of salt

5 glasses of vegetable broth

DIRECTIONS (PREP + COOK TIME: 15 MINUTES)

Boil broth and salt on sear/ sauté mode. Add the polenta flour and stir. Close the pressure lid and cook o high mode for 8 minutes. Quick release the accumulated steam and open the Foodi's lid. Whisk the polenta mixture to smoothen and transfer the meal into serving plates.

Crust-less Quiche

INGREDIENTS (2 Servings)

1/2 cup of Kalamata olives, chopped

4 eggs 1/4 cup of onions, chopped

1/2 cup of milk

1/2 cup of tomatoes, chopped

1 cup of crumbled feta cheese

1 tablespoon of basil, chopped

1 tablespoon of oregano, chopped

2 tablespoons of extra-virgin olive oil

Salt and pepper

DIRECTIONS (PREP + COOK TIME: 40 MINUTES)

Smear the multi-cooker pot with organic olive oil. Beat the eggs into a bowl and add milk. Stir well and season with pepper and salt. Add the remaining ingredients and mix thoroughly. Pour the mixture into the oiled pot and close the crisping lid. Select the Air Crisp button and cook for 30 minutes at 325°F. Cool and serve.

Coconut Scramble

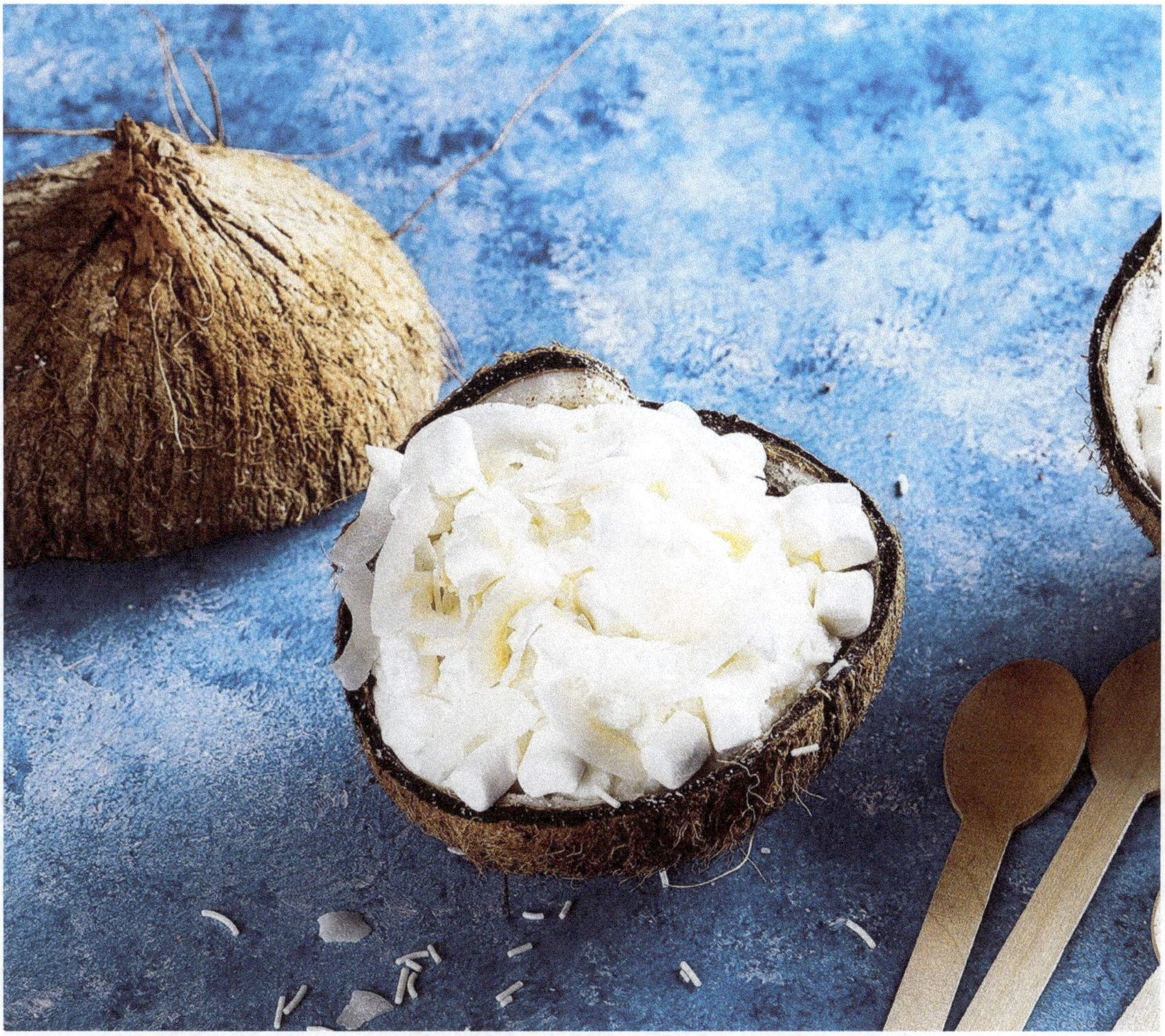

INGREDIENTS (4 Servings)

4 eggs 4 tablespoons of coconut milk

1 red onion, chopped finely

1 tablespoon of canola or coconut oil

4 tablespoons of chives

4 tablespoons of grated cheddar cheese

DIRECTIONS (PREP + COOK TIME: 25 MINUTES)

Press the sauté button on the Foodi multi-cooker. Add the oil and heat it. Add the chopped onions and stir. Sauté the contents for 3 minutes. Combine the remaining ingredients in a bowl and stir. Pour the mixture into the browned onion and toss. Press the air crisp button and cook for 10 minutes (stir after 5 minutes of cooking.) Serve the scramble while hot.

Almond and Berries Cut Oats

INGREDIENTS (4 Servings)

1 cup of cut oats

1 ½ cups of almond milk

½ cup of water

3 tablespoons of maple syrup

1 cup of mixed berries

¼ cup almonds, sliced

1 teaspoon of vanilla flavoring

DIRECTIONS (PREP + COOK TIME: 10 MINUTES)

Combine all the ingredients and close the pressure lid. Cook them for 5 minutes. Release pressure naturally for ten minutes and quick release the remaining steam. Serve the oat breakfast while hot.

Sourdough Bread

INGREDIENTS (1 Servings)

1 ½ cups of water, divided

1 ½ teaspoons of dry yeast

1 teaspoon of sugar

1 cup of plain Greek yogurt

3 cups of all-purpose flour

2 teaspoons of kosher salt

Cooking spray

DIRECTIONS (PREP + COOK TIME: 55 MINUTES)

Add yeast and sugar to a half cup of hot water and stir. Stir the sugary water for 5 minutes or until it becomes foamy. Add flour, yoghurt, and salt to the foamy mixture and mix for 2 minutes using a high-speed mixer. Preheat the multi-cooker for a minute and set it to bake/ roast mode at 250F. Shape the dough into a ball and leave it covered (in the pot) for two hours or until it rises. Place a parchment paper on the reversible rack and grease it with the cooking spray. Transfer the risen dough to the greased paper and shape it into a ball. Cover it with a towel and set aside for 15 minutes. Subdivide the dough into 4″ pieces of ½″ depth approximately. Pour the remaining water into the pot and insert the rack (containing the risen dough) in the Foodi. Close the crisping lid and set the multi-cooker to roast mode. Set the temperatures to 325° F and cook time to 40 minutes. After the bread is cooked, remove it from the rack and let it rest for two hours before serving.

Cheesy Meat Oatmeal

INGREDIENTS (2 Servings)

1 beef sausage, chopped

3 oz. of salami, chopped

4 slices of chopped prosciutto

1 tablespoon of ketchup

1 cup of mozzarella cheese, grated

4 eggs

1 tablespoon of chopped onion

DIRECTIONS (PREP + COOK TIME: 22 MINUTES)

Preheat your Ninja Foodi on 300°F. Set it to Air Crisp mode. Whisk the egg in a bowl. Add the ketchup and whisk. Add the onion and stir again. Grease the Foodi basket with the cooking spray. Add the sausage and cook them for two minutes or until they turn brown. Meanwhile, mix the egg mixture with the chopped salami, mozzarella cheese, and prosciutto. Pour the mixture over the sausage and stir. Close the crisping lid and let it cook for 10 minutes. Serve your meat oatmeal hot.

Breakfast Burritos

INGREDIENTS (4 Servings)

½ cup of milk

8 large eggs

¼ teaspoon of black pepper

½ teaspoon of kosher salt

1 tablespoon of extra virgin olive oil

5 oz. of fresh Mexican chorizo

1 cup of yellow onion, chopped

1 cup of poblano Chile, chopped

½ cup of water

4 ounces (about 1 cup) of Mexican cheese, blend

4 large flour tortillas

½ cup of Pico de Gallo

½ cup of fresh cilantro leaves, loosely packed

DIRECTIONS (PREP + COOK TIME: 40 MINUTES)

Mix the eggs with milk in a bowl. Add salt and pepper. Stir. Preheat the Foodi on sauté mode and cook the chorizo in oil for 5 minutes or until they brown. Add onions and poblano. Cook while stirring frequently for 5 minutes or until they tenders. Stop the sauté mode. Place the chorizo mixture on a foil-lined pan. Pour water into the Ninja Foodi and put the pan in the reversible rack. Spread the egg mixture over the chorizo mixture. Sprinkle the contents with cheese evenly. Insert the rack in the Foodi and close the pressure lid. Cook the mixture on high mode for 20 minutes. Quick release the pressure and open the pressure lid. Place tortillas on a flat surface and subdivide the egg/sausage mixture among them. Top up with two teaspoons of Pico de Gallo and two teaspoons of cilantro. Fold the tortillas' sides and roll up. Enjoy.

Maple Giant Pancake

INGREDIENTS (6 Servings)

3 cups of flour

1/2 cup of essential olive oil

1/3 cup of water

5 eggs

3/4 cup of sugar

2 tablespoon of maple syrup

1 and ½ teaspoon of baking soda

½ teaspoon of salt

A dollop of whipped cream

DIREcTIONS (PREP + COOK TIME: 35 MINUTES)

Mix the flour, eggs, sugar, water, baking soda, and salt in a bowl. Use the mixer to blend it. Pour the mixture into the Ninja Foodi and let it rest for 15 minutes. Close the lid and seal the pressure release valve. Press the pressure cook button and cook on low mode for 10 minutes. Quick release the pressure and open the lid carefully. Remove the pancake using a spatula and place it on a platter. Spread your giant pancake with maple syrup. Serve it with whipped cream toppings.

Air Fried Breakfast Sausage

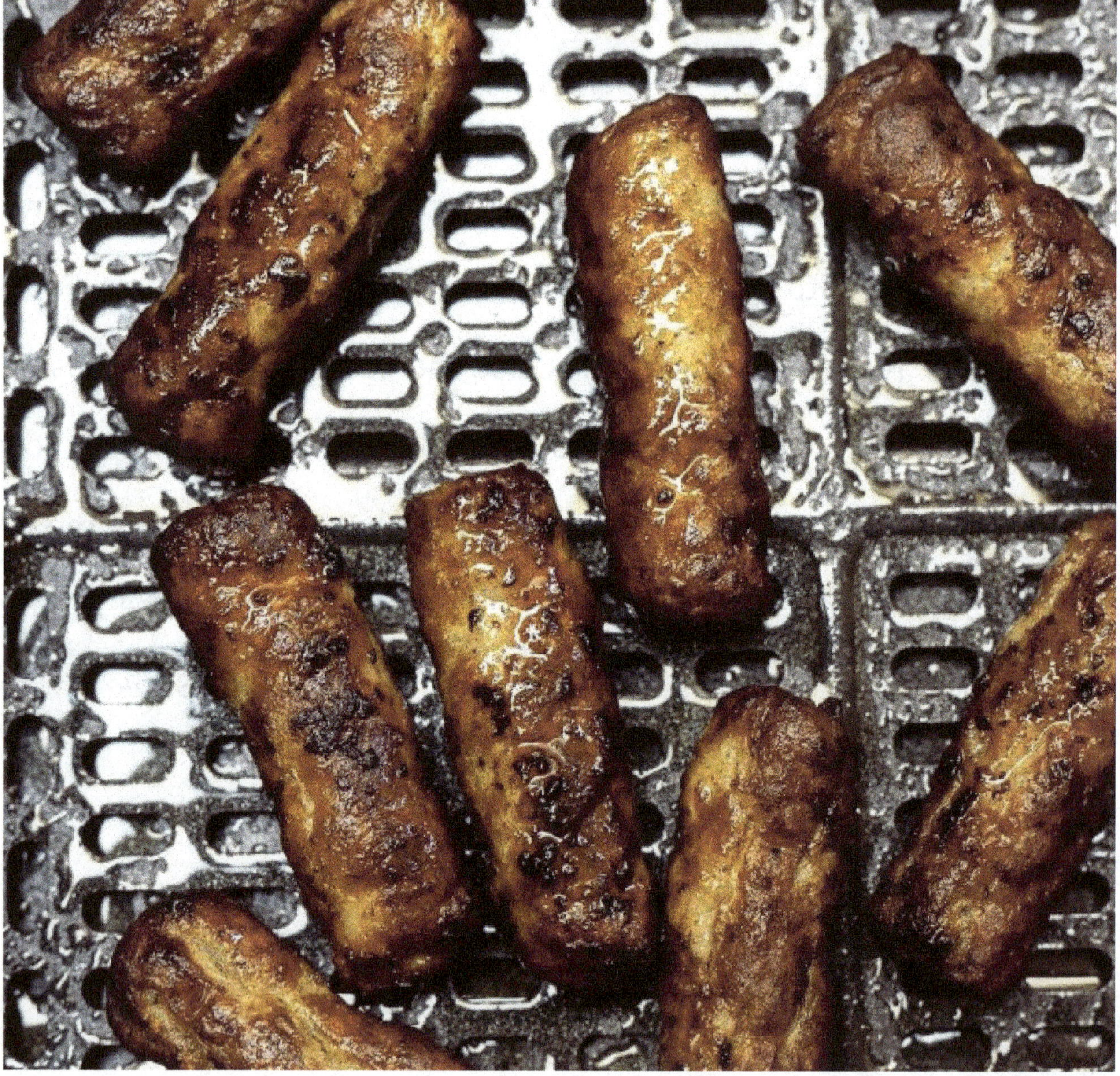

INGREDIENTS (4 Servings)

4 medium sausages

1 teaspoon of celery salt

1 teaspoon of garlic powder

1 egg

DIRECTIONS (PREP + COOK TIME: 15 MINUTES)

Chop the sausages into mince. Add egg, celery salt, and garlic powder to the minced sausages. Form 4 patties and put them in the air crisp basket. Close the crisping lid and press the press crisp function. Set the temperature to 350°F and timer for ten minutes. Select the start/ stop button. Remove the breakfast sausage and serve.

Corned Beef Hash

INGREDIENTS (6 Servings)

1/2 lb of cooked corned beef, diced

2 tablespoons of canola oil

1 red bell pepper, chopped

1 onion (peeled and chopped)

2 medium white potatoes (peeled and diced)

3 teaspoons of salt, divided

1/2 teaspoon of ground black pepper

6 eggs

DIRECTIONS (PREP + COOK TIME: 50 MINUTES)

Sauté the corned beef. Add oil, onion, and potatoes to it. Add 2 teaspoons of salt and pepper. Sauté the seasonings until the onions brown. Cook for 5 minutes or until a crust forms at the bottom while stirring frequently. Cook for five more minutes and stir. Crack the eggs over the potatoes and close the crisping lid. Broil for 10 minutes. Serve the beef hash with hot sauce. You can also garnish with parsley.

Gold Potatoes and Bacon

INGREDIENTS (8 Servings)

2 gold potatoes, cubed

8 oz. of bacon, chopped

4 eggs, beaten

1 red bell pepper, chopped

1 yellow onion, chopped

Salt and black pepper

1 teaspoon of sweet paprika

DIRECTIONS (PREP + COOK TIME: 50 MINUTES)

Set the Foodi to sauté mode. Add the bacon and cook for 5 minutes. Add the bell pepper, onions, and gold potatoes. Sauté the mixture for 5 more minutes. Add eggs, paprika, salt, and black pepper. Set the Foodi to air fry mode and close the crisping lid. Cook the contents for thirty minutes at a temperature of 300°F. Remember to flip at around 15 minutes. Serve hot.

Simple Corned Beef Hash

INGREDIENTS (6 Servings)

2 medium cans of corned beef, diced

12 white potatoes, medium- sized

4 large carrots

1 large white onion

1and ½ cups of beef stock

1 teaspoon of parsley

Salt and pepper

DIRECTIONS (PREP + COOK TIME: 13 MINUTES)

Dice the corn beef and set aside. Prepare the vegetables by dicing the carrots, potatoes, and onions. Put the diced veggies in the Foodi and add the beef stock. Close the pressure lid on and seal the pressure valve. Cook at high mode for ten minutes. Quick release the pressure when the cooking time elapses. Open the lid and add salt and pepper. Add the diced beef and set the multi-cooker to Sauté mode. Let it cook for two minutes and serve hot.

Tuna Bowls

INGREDIENTS (4 Servings)

16 oz. of canned tuna (drained and flaked)

1 red onion, chopped

½ cup of baby spinach

2 spring onions, chopped

1 tablespoons of lime juice

3 tablespoons of melted butter

DIRECTIONS (PREP + COOK TIME: 13 MINUTES)

Set your Ninja Foodi to sauté mode and preheat it for a minute. Add butter and melt. Add onions to the butter and cook for 2 minutes while stirring. Add the remaining ingredients and stir. Close the pressure lid and set the release valve to seal position. Cook the ingredients for 5 minutes and quick release the accumulated pressure after the cooking time elapses. Subdivide the tuna bowls amongst four plates and enjoy.

Oatmeal with Carrot

INGREDIENTS (6 Servings)

1 tablespoon of butter

1 cup of cut oats

1 cup of carrots, grated

4 cups of water

1 teaspoon of pumpkin pie spice

3 tablespoons of maple syrup

¼ teaspoon of salt

¼ cup of dried apricots, chopped

½ cup of slivered almonds

½ cup of raisins

DIRECTIONS (PREP + COOK TIME: 23 MINUTES)

Put butter into the Foodi and melt it on sauté mode. Add the oats and sauté for 3 minutes while stirring consistently. Add the water, carrots, maple syrup, spices, and salt. Close the pressure lid and set the release valve to "seal." Cook the ingredients on high mode for ten minutes. Let the steam exit naturally for 10 minutes and quick release the rest. Open the pressure lid and add cinnamon, almonds, apricots, and raisins. Stir. Let your oatmeal rest for 5 minutes before serving.

Spicy Tomato Eggs

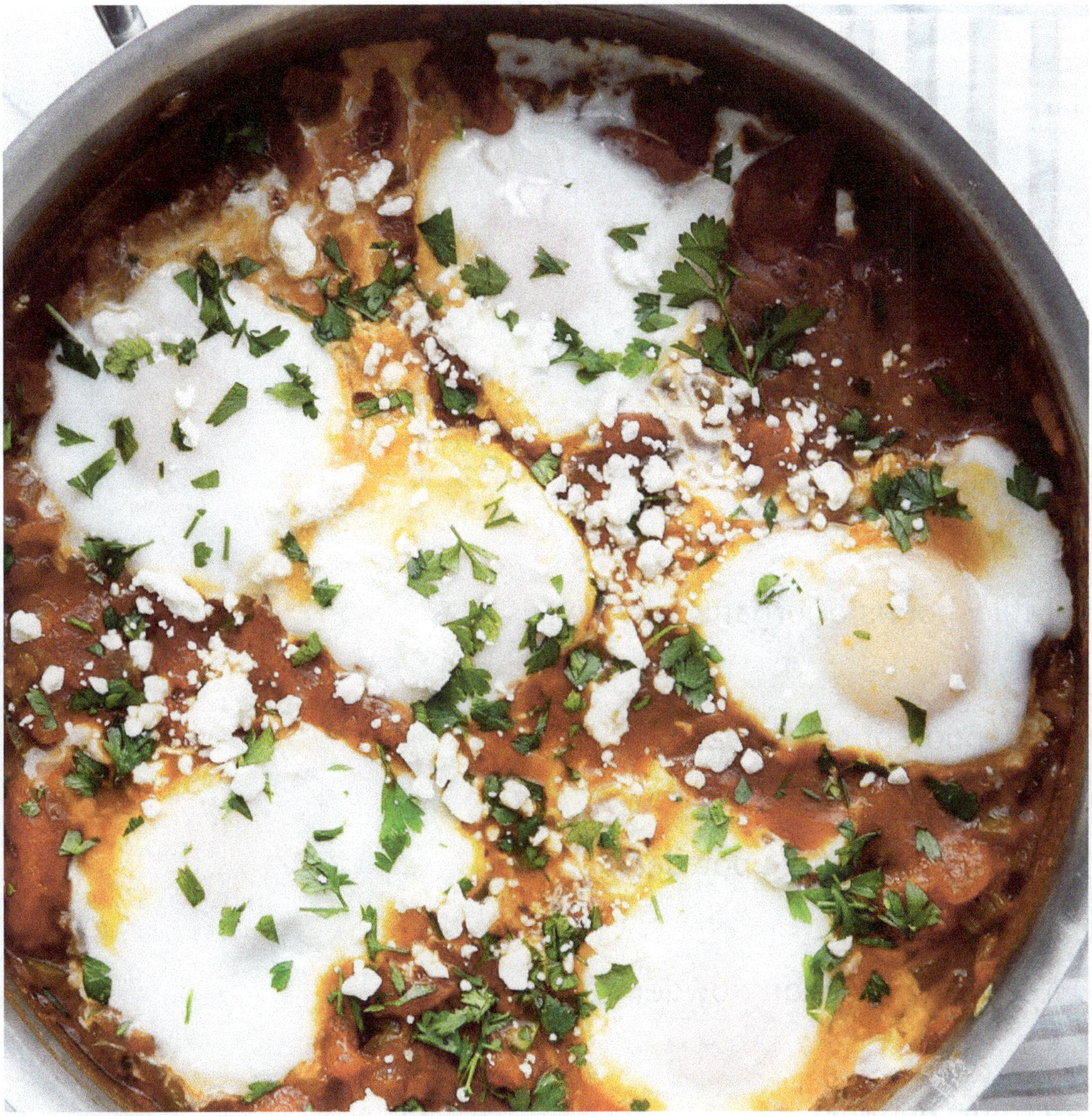

INGREDIENTS (4 Servings)

1 red bell pepper, chopped

2 tomatoes, cubed

4 eggs, whisked

1 yellow onion

2 tablespoons of organic olive oil

1 teaspoon of sweet paprika

1 teaspoon of garlic powder

1 teaspoon of onion powder

Salt and pepper

DIRECTIONS (PREP + COOK TIME: 30 MINUTES)

Set your Foodi to sauté mode and heat some olive oil. Add the bell pepper to the heated oil let it cook for five minutes while stirring occasionally. Add the cubed tomatoes, onion powder, garlic powder, paprika, salt, and pepper. Stir. Cook the ingredients for five more minutes. Add the eggs and toss well. Close the pressure lid and cook on high mode for 12 minutes. Natural-release the accumulated pressure for ten minutes. Subdivide your spiced tomato eggs amongst four plates.

Brown Rice Breakfast Risotto

INGREDIENTS (4 Servings)

2 tablespoons of butter

1 ½ cups of short grain brown rice

2 medium bananas, mashed lightly

1/3 cup of brown sugar

1 ½ teaspoons of cinnamon

½ teaspoon of salt

3 cups of light coconut milk

1 cup of dry white wine

Chopped walnuts

DIRECTIONS (PREP + COOK TIME: 30 MINUTES)

Smear some butter on your Foodi's base and melt it on sauté mode. Add the rice and cook for two minutes while stirring constantly. Add the bananas, cinnamon, salt, sugar, milk, and wine. Close the pressure lid and cook on high mode for 22 minutes. Natural-release the in-built pressure and serve with chopped walnuts garnishing.

Turkey Burrito

INGREDIENTS (2 Servings)

1 turkey breast (cooked and shredded)

3 eggs, whisked

1 red pepper, sliced

1 avocado (peeled, pitted, and sliced)

Salt and pepper

2 tablespoons of shredded mozzarella cheese

2 corn tortillas

Cooking spray

DIRECTIONS (PREP + COOK TIME: 11 MINUTES)

Smear the pan with the cooking spray. Add salt, pepper, and the whisked eggs into a pan and mix. Add the remaining ingredients except cheese and tortilla. Whisk well. Fix the reversible rack in the pot and place a pan on it. Cover the pan's content with a foil and closes the pressure lid. Cook on high mode for10 minutes and then quick release the accumulated steam. Place the tortillas on a clean surface and subdivide the egg mixture equally amongst them. Top each of them with mozzarella cheese and enjoy

Cauliflower Mix

INGREDIENTS (4 Servings)

1 ½ cups of white cauliflower, florets separated

1 ½ cups of purple cauliflower, florets separated

2 garlic cloves, minced.

½ cup of peas

1 carrot, cubed.

2 spring onions, chopped

2 and ½ teaspoons of soy sauce

2 teaspoons of organic olive oil

A pinch of salt and black pepper

DIRECTIONS (PREP + COOK TIME: 20 MINUTES)

Set the Foodi to Sauté mode and add oil. Heat it up. Add the onions and garlic and stir. Cook for three minutes. Add the carrots, cauliflower, soy sauce, salt, pepper, and peas. Toss and close the pressure lid. Cook on high mode for 8 minutes. Release the pressure naturally for ten minutes. Subdivide your cauliflower mix between plates as a side dish.

Potato Salad

INGREDIENTS (6 Servings)

2 lb of red potatoes, scrubbed

1 yellow onion, chopped

5 bacon strips, chopped

2 celery stalks, chopped

¼ cup of apple cider vinegar

1 cup of sauerkraut

½ cup of scallions, chopped

½ cup of water

1 tablespoon of mustard

¼ teaspoon of sweet paprika

1 teaspoon of sugar

A pinch of salt and black pepper

DIRECTIONS (PREP + COOK TIME: 25 MINUTES)

Put the potatoes and water into the Ninja Foodi and close the pressure lid. Cook on high mode for 5 minutes and release the pressure naturally for 10 minutes Cool the potatoes, peel, and cube them. Clean the Foodi and set it to sauté mode. Add the bacon and stir. Cook for 5 minutes Add the onions and stir. Cook for another 5 minutes. Add vinegar and toss. Cook for one minute. Add the scrubbed potatoes and the remaining ingredients. Toss and cook until the potatoes soften. Subdivide your potato salad between plates as a side dish.

Garlicky Broccoli

INGREDIENTS (4 Servings)

1 broccoli head, florets separated

3 garlic cloves, minced

2 tablespoons of lemon juice

2 tablespoons of parsley, chopped

1 tablespoon of essential olive oil

DIRECTIONS (PREP + COOK TIME: 30 MINUTES)

Set the Foodi on sauté mode and add oil. Heat it up. Add the garlic, broccoli, and lemon juice. Toss and cook for two minutes Close the pressure lid and cook on high mode for 15 minutes. Let the accumulated pressure release for 10 minutes naturally. Subdivide your garlicky broccoli between serving plates as a side dish.

Easy Gnocchi

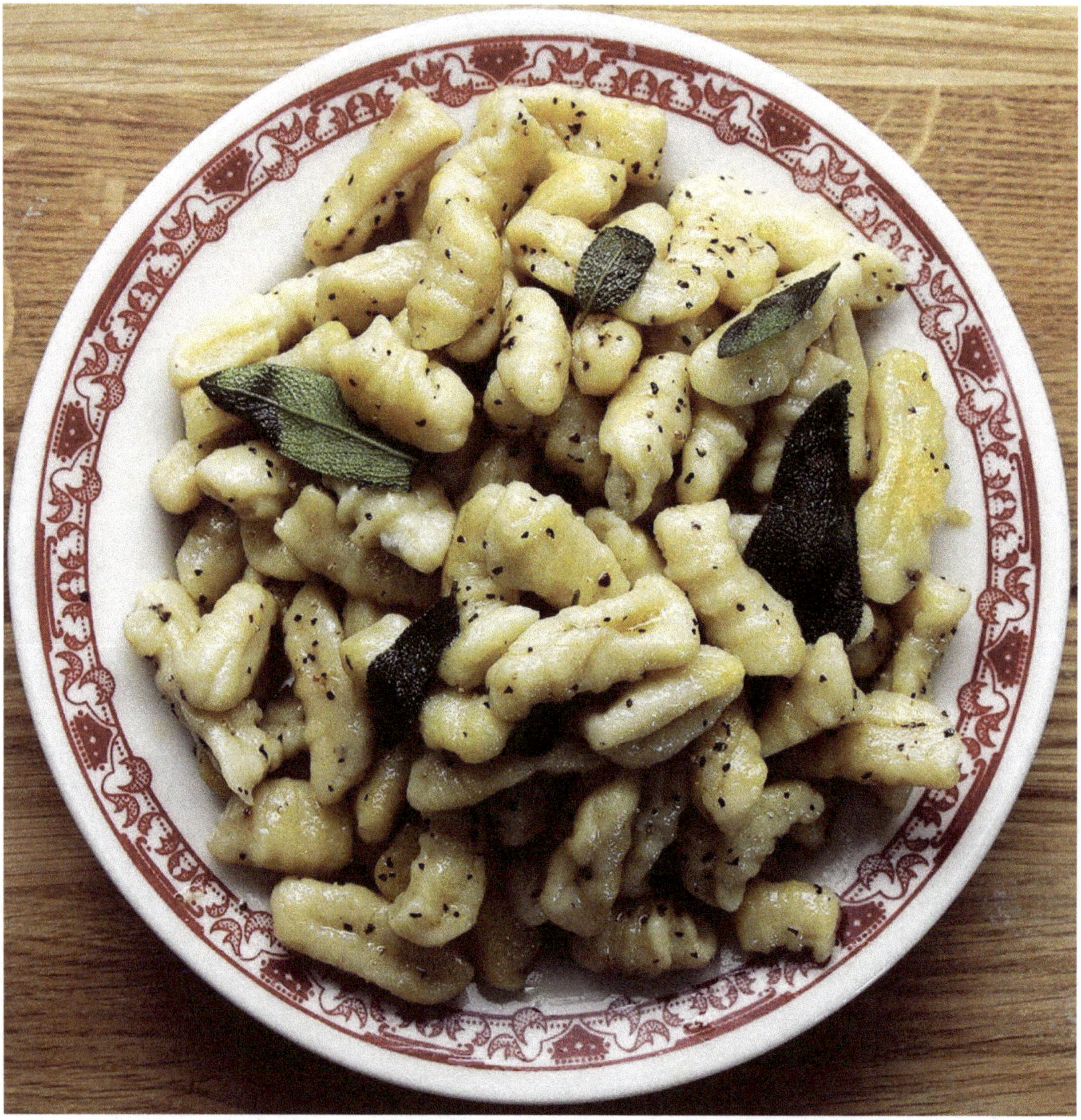

INGREDIENTS (6 Servings)

50 oz. of potato gnocchi

10 oz. of baby spinach

½ cup of goat cheese, crumbled

¼ cup of parmesan, grated

1/3 cup of white flour

3 and ½ cups of heavy cream

1 ½ cups of chicken stock

A pinch of salt and black pepper

DIRECTIONS (PREP + COOK TIME: 32 MINUTES)

Set the Foodi to Sauté mode and heat it up. Add the stock, cream, flour, salt, pepper, and nutmeg. Whisk well and cook for 8 minutes. Add the spinach and gnocchi. Sprinkle the mixture with parmesan and goat cheese. Set the Foodi to bake mode and cook at 325 °F for 15 minutes. Subdivide your gnocchi side dish amongst plates.

Warm Potato Salad

INGREDIENTS (4 Servings)

2 gold potatoes cut into wedges

3 tablespoons of heavy cream

1 tablespoon of canola oil

Salt and black pepper

DIRECTIONS (PREP + COOK TIME: 30 MINUTES)

Put the potatoes in the air crisp basket and insert it in the Foodi. Set the multi-cooker to air crisp mode and cook at 400 °F for 10 minutes Transfer the potatoes to a bowl and clean the

Foodi. Set it to sauté mode and add oil. Heat it up. Put the potato wedges, salt, pepper, and cream into the pot. Toss and cook for 10 minutes. Subdivide your salad between plates as a side dish

Zucchini Fries

INGREDIENTS (4 Servings)

2 small zucchinis cut into fries

2 eggs, whisked

1 cup of bread crumbs

½ cup of white flour

Cooking spray

Salt and black pepper

DIRECTIONS (PREP + COOK TIME: 22 MINUTES)

Mix flour, salt, and pepper in a bowl. Stir. Put the breadcrumbs in another bowl and add the whisked eggs. Dredge the zucchini fries in the bread crumb mixture and transfer them to the Foodi's air crisp basket. Fix the basket in the Foodi and grease the fries with the cooking spray. Set the multi-cooker to air crisp mode and cook at 400 °F for 12 minutes. Subdivide your zucchini side dish between plates.

Veggie Side Salad

INGREDIENTS (4 Servings)

1 eggplant, cubed

1 green bell pepper, chopped

1 bunch of cilantro, chopped

2 garlic cloves, minced

1 yellow onion, chopped

1 tablespoon of tomato sauce

1 tablespoon of extra virgin olive oil

Salt and black pepper

DIRECTIONS (PREP + COOK TIME: 22 MINUTES)

Set the Foodi to Sauté mode and add the oil. Heat it up. Add all the ingredients (except the cilantro) and toss. Close the pressure lid and cook on high mode for 12 minutes. Release pressure naturally for 10 minutes. Subdivide your veggie side dish between plates and enjoy.

Sumac Eggplant

INGREDIENTS (6 Servings)

2 lb of eggplants, cubed

1 tablespoon of organic olive oil

1 teaspoon of sumac

1 teaspoon of garlic powder

Juice extracted from a lime.

DIRECTIONS (PREP + COOK TIME: 25 MINUTES)

Set the Foodi to sauté mode and add oil. Heat it up. Add the eggplant, garlic powder, sumac, and lime juice. Toss and close the pressure lid. Cook on high mode for 15 minutes. Release the pressure for 10 minutes naturally. Subdivide the eggplant mixture between plates as a side dish.

Thyme Red Potatoes

INGREDIENTS (4 Servings)

4 red potatoes, thinly sliced

1 tablespoon of organic olive oil

2 teaspoons of thyme, chopped

Salt and black pepper

DIRECTIONS (PREP + COOK TIME: 40 MINUTES)

Mix all the ingredients in a bowl and toss. Transfer the mixture to an air crisp basket and insert it in the Foodi. Set the multi-cooker to air crisp mode and cook at 370 °F for 30 minutes. Subdivide your thyme-potatoes between serving plates as a side dish

Cauliflower and Pineapple Salad

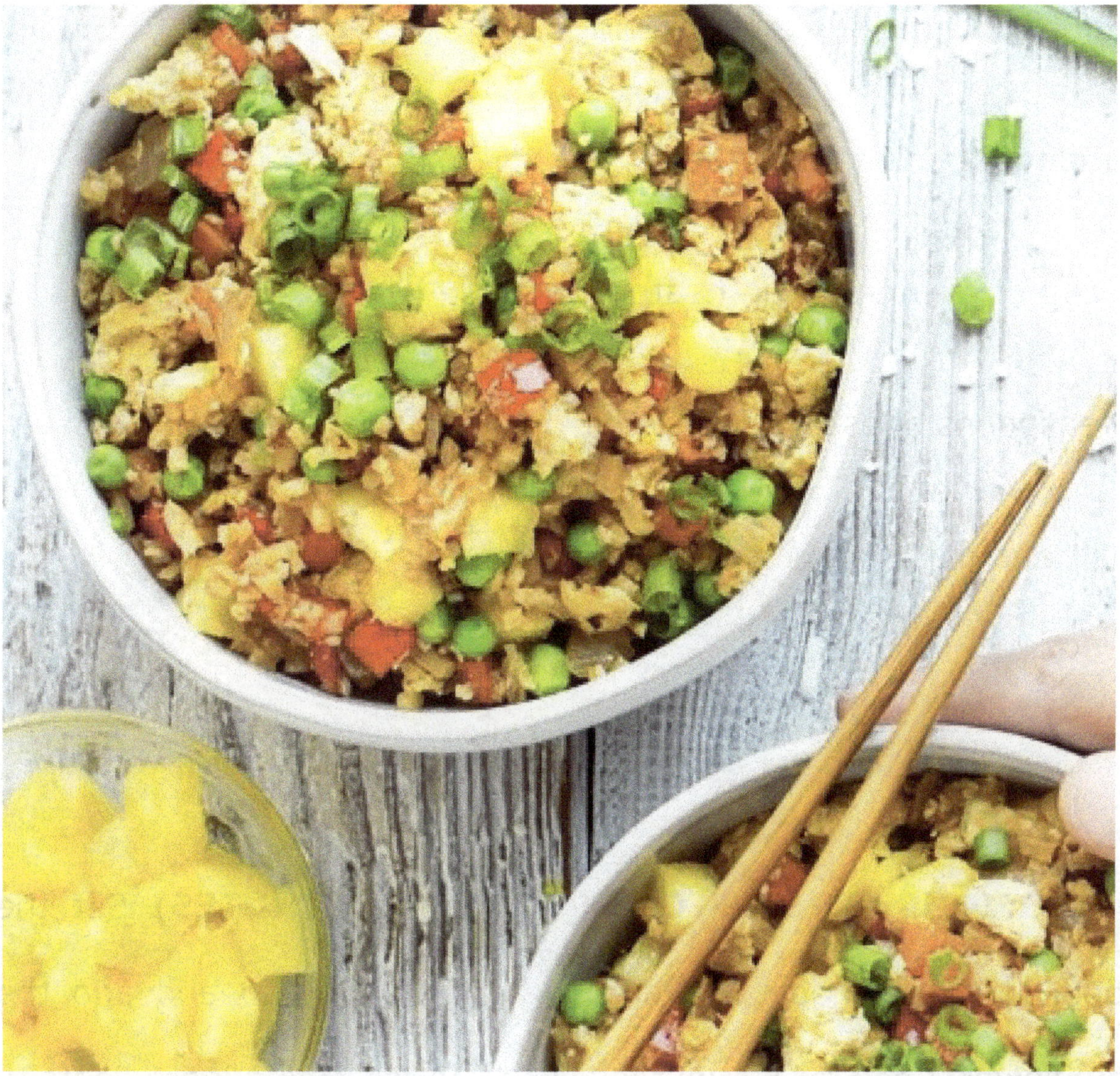

INGREDIENTS (6 Servings)

2 cauliflower florets

1 pineapple (peeled and cubed)

1 mango (peeled and cubed)

1 cup of chicken stock, heated up

2 teaspoons of essential olive oil

Salt and black pepper

DIRECTIONS (PREP + COOK TIME: 30 MINUTES) Set the Foodi to sauté mode and add the oil. Heat it up and add the cauliflower. Cook for 5 minutes. Add the remaining ingredients to the pot and close the pressure lid. Cook on high mode for 15 minutes and release the steam naturally for 10 minutes. Subdivide your pineapple salad between serving plates as a side dish.

Hazelnut Cauliflower Rice

INGREDIENTS (4 Servings)

1 spring onion, chopped

2 garlic cloves, minced

2 cups of cauliflower rice

2 cups of chicken stock

½ cup of hazelnuts (toasted and chopped)

1 tablespoon of cilantro (chopped)

1 teaspoon of essential olive oil

Salt and black pepper

DIRECTIONS (PREP + COOK TIME: 32 MINUTES)

Set the Foodi to Sauté mode and add the oil. Warm it and add onions. Add the minced garlic and stir. Cook for 3 minutes. Add the cauliflower rice, stock, hazelnuts, salt, and pepper. Toss and close the pressure lid. Cook on high mode for 20 minutes. Release the accumulated steam naturally for 10 minutes. Add the chopped cilantro and toss. Subdivide your cauliflower rice between serving plates as a side dish.

Maple Carrots

INGREDIENTS (6 Servings)

2 lbs of carrots, roughly cubed

1 tablespoon of canola oil

2 tablespoon of maple syrup

1 tablespoon of parsley, chopped

DIRECTIONS (PREP + COOK TIME: 25 MINUTES)

Mix all the ingredients in a bowl and transfer the mixture into an air crisp basket. Fit the basket in the Foodi and set it to crisping mode. Cook at 350 °F for 20 minutes. Subdivide the maple carrots between serving plates as a side dish.

Green Beans Salad

INGREDIENTS (4 Servings)

1 ½ lb of green beans, trimmed

½ lb of shallots, chopped

¼ cup of walnuts, chopped

2 tablespoons of olive oil

Salt and black pepper

DIRECTIONS (PREP + COOK TIME: 30 MINUTES)

Combine all the ingredients in the crisping basket and fix it in the Foodi Set the multi-cooker to air crisp mode and cook at 360 °F for 20 minutes. Subdivide your beans' salad between serving plates as a side dish.

Roasted Tomato Salad

INGREDIENTS (2 Servings)

20 oz. of cherry tomatoes, cut into quarters

½ cup of cilantro

1 white onion, roughly chopped

1 jalapeno pepper, chopped

Juice extracted from one lime

1 tablespoon of extra virgin olive oil

Salt and black pepper

DIRECTIONS (PREP + COOK TIME: 16 MINUTES)

Set the Foodi to sauté mode and add the oil. Heat it and add the onions. Stir and sauté the onions for three minutes. Add the remaining ingredients and toss. Set the Ninja Foodi to roast mode and cook at 380 °F for 4 minutes. Subdivide your tomato salad between serving plates as a side dish.

Potato Mash

INGREDIENTS (4 Servings)

3 gold potatoes (peeled and cubed)

½ cup of cheddar cheese, shredded

1 cup of heavy cream

1 cup of water

¼ cup of butter, melted

A pinch of salt and black pepper

DIRECTIONS (PREP + COOK TIME: 20 MINUTES)

Put the potatoes and water in the Foodi and close the pressure lid. Cook on high mode for ten minutes and release the pressure naturally for another ten minutes. Drain the potatoes and transfer them to a bowl. Mash them and add butter, cheese, cream, salt, and pepper. Stir. Subdivide your potato mash between serving plates as a side dish.

Spiced Squash

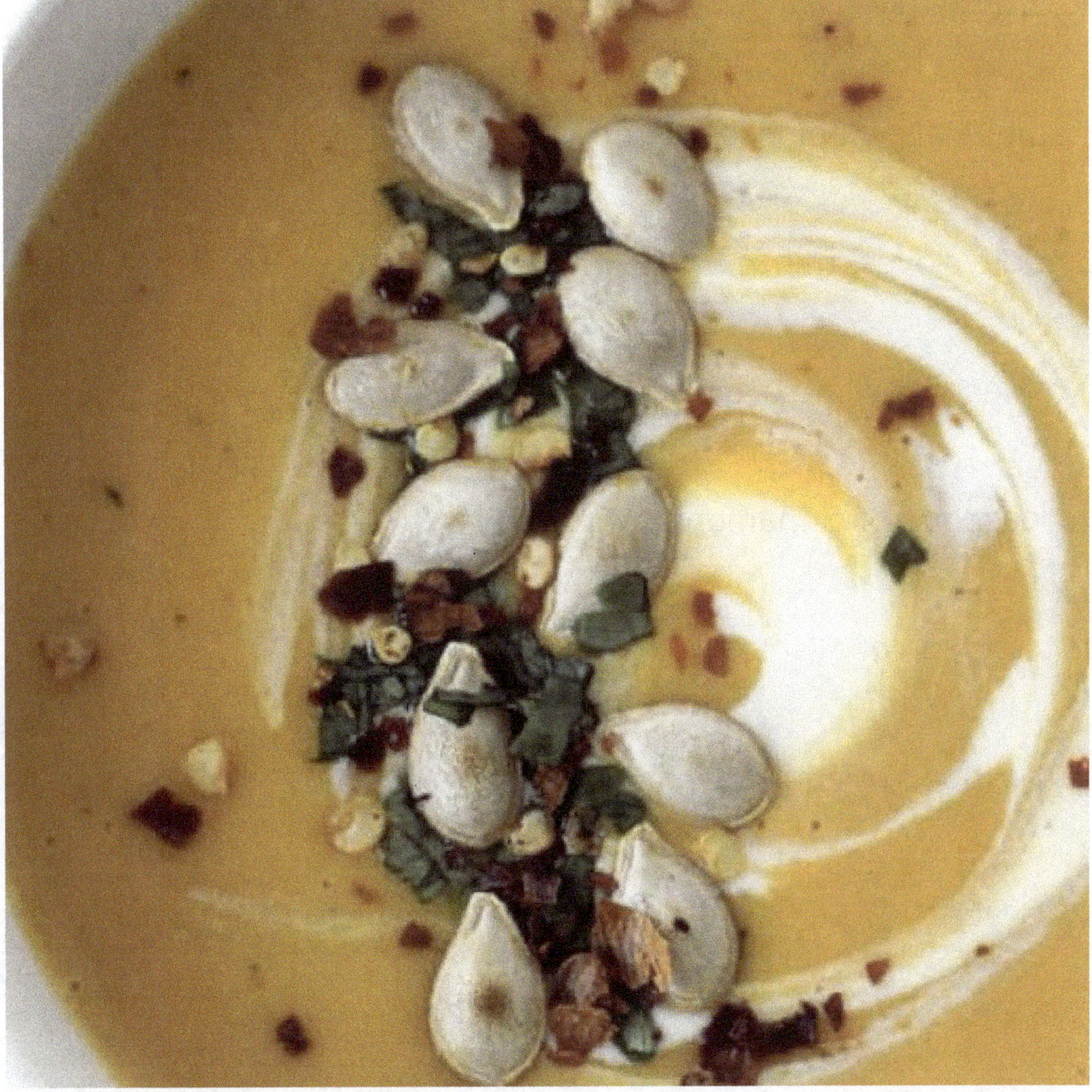

INGREDIENTS (4 Servings)

6 oz of squash, cubed

2 oz of heavy cream

1 small yellow onion, chopped

2 garlic cloves, minced

2 tablespoons of extra virgin olive oil

½ teaspoon of cinnamon powder

½ teaspoon of allspice

½ teaspoon of nutmeg, ground

½ teaspoon of ginger, grated

DIRECTIONS (PREP + COOK TIME: 25 MINUTES)

Set the Foodi to sauté mode and add the oil. Heat it up. Add onions and garlic. Stir and cook for 5 minutes. Add the remaining ingredients and toss. Set the Foodi to baking mode and cook everything at 360 °F for fifteen minutes. Subdivide your squash between serving plates as a side dish.

Beans and Tomatoes Mix

INGREDIENTS (6 Servings)

1 lb of canned red kidney beans, drained

½ lb of cherry tomatoes, cut into quarters

1 yellow onion, chopped

4 garlic cloves, chopped

2 spring onions, minced

1 teaspoon of essential olive oil

2 tablespoons of cilantro, minced

2 tablespoons of tomato sauce

Salt and black pepper

DIRECTIONS (PREP + COOK TIME: 30 MINUTES)

Mix all the ingredients (except cilantro) in your Foodi's baking pan and toss. Insert the reversible rack in the equipment and place the baking pan on it. Set the Foodi to baking mode and cook everything for 20 minutes. Add the minced cilantro and stir. Subdivide your tomatoes side dish between plates and enjoy.

Potatoes and Tomatoes

INGREDIENTS (6 Servings)

15 oz of potatoes, cubed

6 oz of canned tomatoes, chopped

2 spring onions, chopped

2 tablespoons of extra virgin olive oil

½ teaspoon of nutmeg, ground

Salt and black pepper

DIRECTIONS (PREP + COOK TIME: 25 MINUTES)

Set the Foodi to sauté mode and add the oil. Heat it up and add the onions. Stir and cook for 3 minutes. Add the potatoes, nutmeg, tomatoes, salt, and pepper to the onions. Toss and close the pressure lid. Cook on high mode for fifteen minutes. Release the accumulated vapor naturally for ten minutes. Subdivide the side dish between plates and enjoy.

Creamy Cauliflower

INGREDIENTS (4 Servings)

1 cauliflower head, florets separated

½ cup of Italian bread crumbs

¼ cup of raisins

½ cup of heavy cream

½ cup of parmesan, grated

1 cup of beer

1 tablespoon of white flour

A teaspoon of nutmeg, ground

A pinch of salt and black pepper

DIRECTIONS (PREP + COOK TIME: 25 MINUTES)

Combine beer with the raisins, cauliflower, salt, pepper, and nutmeg in your Foodi. Toss and close the pressure lid. Cook the ingredients on high mode for 3 minutes. Release the pressure naturally for four minutes and quick release the rest. Add the cream mixed with the flour and toss. Set the Foodi to sauté mode and continue cooking for 5 more minutes. Mix the bread crumbs with cheese in a bowl. Stir and pour it over the cauliflower mixture. Close the crisping lid and set the Foodi to air crisp mode. Cook at 390 °F for ten minutes. Subdivide your creamy cauliflower between serving plates as a side dish.

Garlic Mushrooms

INGREDIENTS (4 Servings)

1 lb of brown mushrooms, halved

1 tablespoon of garlic, minced

A tablespoon of lime juice

1 tablespoon of chives, chopped

2 tablespoons of extra virgin olive oil

Salt and black pepper

DIRECTIONS (PREP + COOK TIME: 30 MINUTES)

Set the Foodi to sauté mode and add the oil. Warm it and add garlic and mushrooms. Toss and sauté for 5 minutes Add the lime juice and set the multi-cooker to baking mode. Cook at 380 °F for 15 minutes. Add the chives and toss. Subdivide the mushroom side dish between serving plates and enjoy.

Sweet Potato and Mayo

INGREDIENTS (2 Servings)

2 sweet potatoes (peeled and cut into wedges)

4 tablespoons of mayonnaise

2 tablespoons of organic olive oil

½ teaspoon of curry powder

¼ teaspoon of coriander, ground

½ teaspoon of cumin, ground

A pinch of ginger powder

Salt and black pepper

DIRECTIONS (PREP + COOK TIME: 30 MINUTES)

Mix the sweet potato wedges with salt, pepper, coriander, curry powder, and oil in the crisping basket. Toss well. Insert the basket in the Foodi and set it to air crisp mode. Cook the potatoes at 380 °F for 20 minutes. Remember to shake the pot at the 10th minute. Transfer the potatoes to a bowl and add the remaining ingredients. Toss and serve as a side dish.

Yummy Eggplant

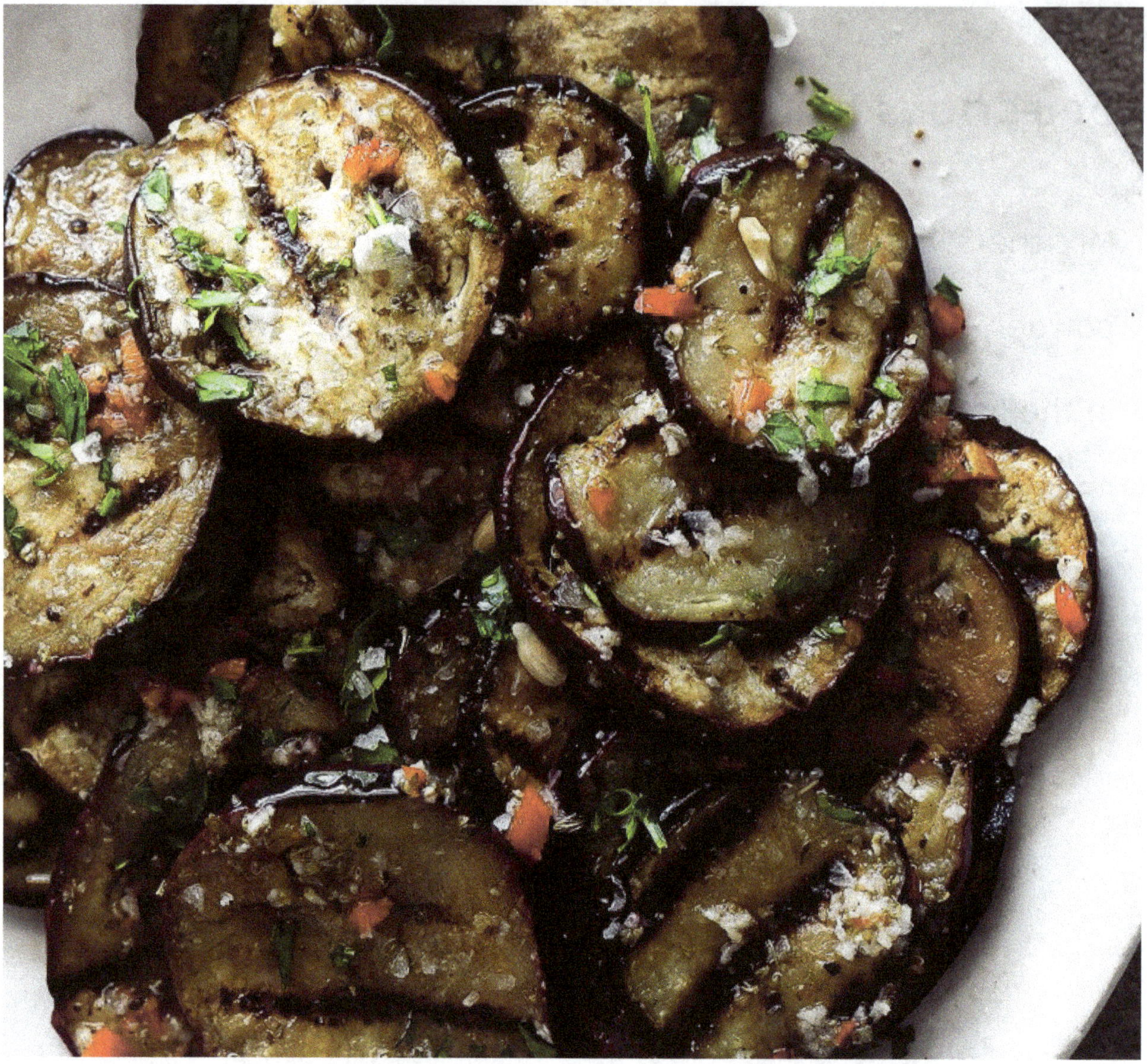

INGREDIENTS (4 Servings)

4 eggplants (cut into cubes)

1 red onion, chopped

1 tablespoon of smoked paprika

1 tablespoon of organic olive oil

Salt and black pepper

DIRECTIONS (PREP + COOK TIME: 25 MINUTES)

Set the Foodi to Sauté mode and add the oil. Heat it up and add the eggplants followed by the remaining ingredients. Stir. Close the pressure lid and cook on high mode for fifteen minutes. Release the pressure naturally for 10 minutes. Subdivide your yummy eggplants between serving plates as a side dish.

Buttery Brussels sprouts

INGREDIENTS (8 Servings)

3 lbs of Brussels sprouts, trimmed

1 lb of bacon, chopped

1 yellow onion, chopped

2 cups of heavy cream

4 tablespoons of butter, melted

1 teaspoon of extra virgin olive oil

Salt and black pepper

DIRECTIONS (PREP + COOK TIME: 30 MINUTES)

Put the Brussels sprouts in the crisping basket and insert it in your Ninja Foodi. Set it to air crisp mode and cook at 370 °F for 10 minutes. Transfer the cooked sprouts to a bowl and clean the Foodi. Set the multi-cooker to sauté mode and add oil and butter. Heat it to melt the butter. Return the sprouts to the Foodi and add the chopped bacon. Add onions and stir. Continue cooking the ingredients for five more minutes. Subdivide the sprouts between plates as a side dish.

Asian Style Chickpeas

INGREDIENTS (4 Servings)

30 oz of canned chickpeas, drained

2 tablespoons of olive oil

2 teaspoons of garam Masala

¼ teaspoon of mustard powder

½ teaspoon of garlic powder

1 teaspoon of sweet paprika

A pinch of salt and black pepper

DIRECTIONS (PREP + COOK TIME: 30 MINUTES)

Mix all the ingredients in a bowl and toss well. Set the Ninja Foodi to sauté mode and heat it up for 3 minutes. Add the chickpeas mixture and sauté them for 6 minutes Transfer them to the Foodi's basket and set it to air crisp mode. Cook the mixture at 400 °F for fifteen minutes. Subdivide your chickpeas side dish between plates as a side dish.

Brussels sprouts

INGREDIENTS (4 Servings)

1 lb of Brussels sprouts, halved

4 bacon strips (cooked and chopped)

1 tablespoon of extra virgin olive oil

2 teaspoons of garlic powder

A pinch of salt and black pepper

DIRECTIONS (PREP + COOK TIME: 25 MINUTES)

Mix all the ingredients in a bowl (except bacon) and toss. Put the Brussels sprouts in the crisping basket and set it to air crisp mode. Cook at 390 °F for twenty minutes. Subdivide the Brussels sprouts between plates and top them with bacon.

Roasted Potatoes

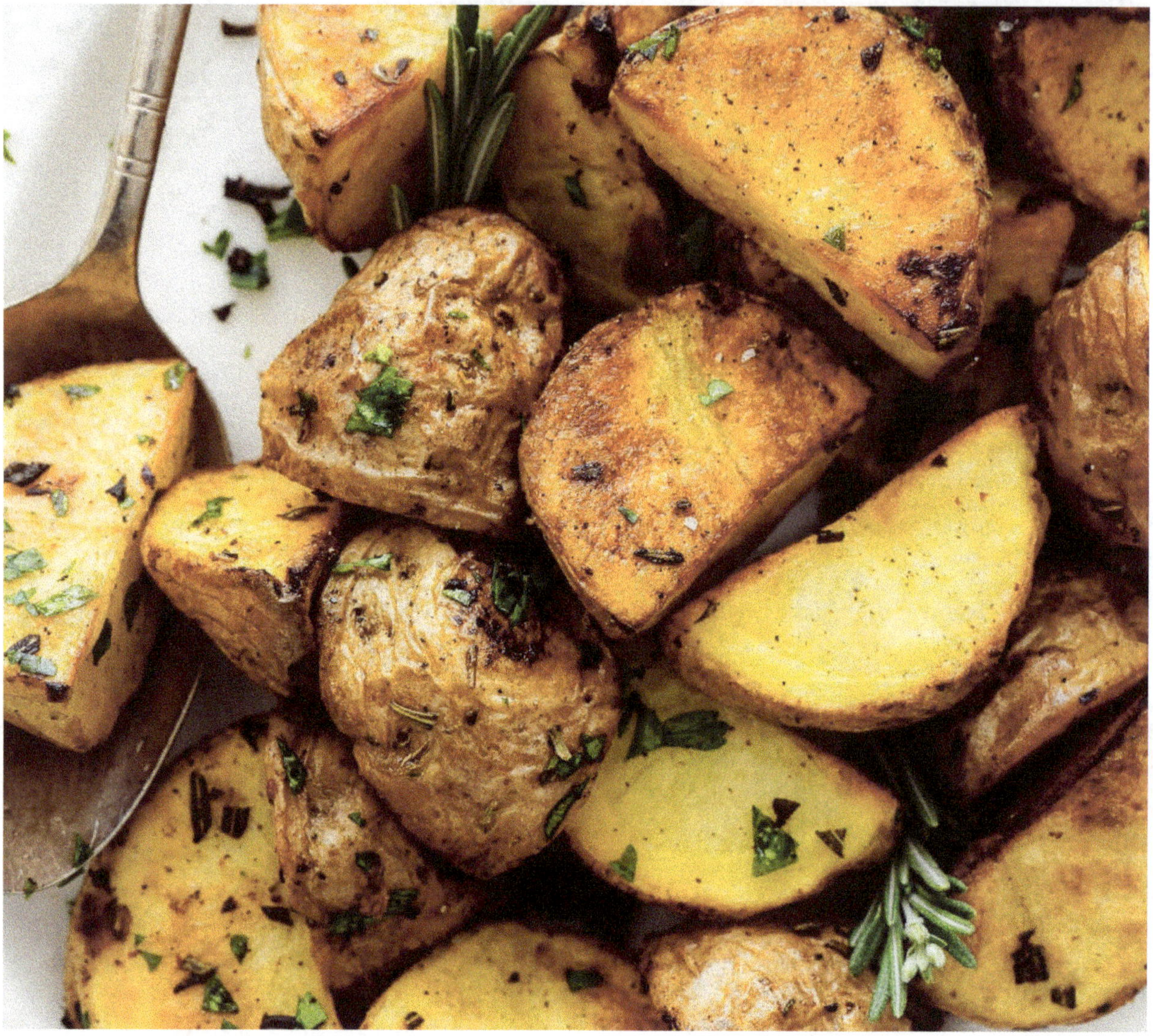

INGREDIENTS (4 Servings)

1 lb of baby potatoes, halved

½ cup of parsley, chopped

½ cup of mayonnaise

2 tablespoons of tomato paste

2 tablespoons of extra virgin olive oil

1 tablespoons of smoked paprika

A tablespoon of garlic powder

2 tablespoons of white wine vinegar

3 teaspoons of hot paprika

A pinch of salt and black pepper

DIRECTIONS (PREP + COOK TIME: 35 MINUTES)

Combine the potatoes with hot paprika, oil, smoked paprika, garlic powder, salt, and pepper in a bowl. Toss well. Put the potatoes in the crisping basket and insert it in the Foodi. Set the multi-cooker to air crisp mode and cook the potatoes at 360 °F for 25 minutes. Transfer the mixture to a bowl and add tomato paste, mayo, vinegar, and parsley. Toss your roasted potatoes and serve as a side dish.

Conclusion

Did you delight in trying these new and scrumptious recipes?

Regrettably we have come to the end of this recipe book regarding the use of the amazing Ninja Foodi multi-cooker, which I truly wish you taken pleasure in.

To improve your wellness we wish to advise you to combine physical activity and a vibrant lifestyle along with following these amazing recipes, so as to highlight the renovations. we will be back quickly with a growing number of appealing vegan recipes, a large hug, see you quickly.

CPSIA information can be obtained
at www.ICGtesting.com
Printed in the USA
LVHW061939180521
687789LV00003B/502